YOGA

Yoga for Busy People

Health, Fitness, and Stress Relief on the Go

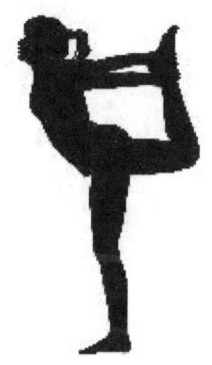

Misty Jordyn

Misty Jordyn

TABLE OF CONTENTS

CHAPTER ONE

WHAT IS YOGA AND WHY SHOULD I PRACTICE IT?

Yoga is a well-known, ancient technique of mediation, spiritual awareness, breathing exercises and physical movements designed to strengthen muscles, reduce stress and increase overall health.

Physically speaking, this looks like a variety of long stretches, gentle movements and deep relaxation of the body and mind.

Don't let this lull you into the idea that it is not "real exercise" however. Seemingly simple exercises can be quite challenging to a novice. With further practice, however, all yoga poses become easier with time.

As modern life becomes more stressful, yoga has become increasingly popular as a way to relieve stress and maintain a healthy balance in life. The good news is that the benefits of yoga begin to show up once you start taking ten to fifteen minutes out of your day. Although it would be nice to spend an hour in meditation, fifteen minutes is plenty. You will find a new sense of self-confidence and peace that will make anything life has to offer easier to handle.

There are five principles of yoga: proper relaxation, proper breathing, proper exercise, proper diet, and positive meditation and thinking.

Proper relaxation is the ability to release the tension in the muscles and allow the entire body to rest. This revitalizes the nervous system and help to maintain inner peace. The relaxed feeling of inner peace carries over into your day to day life and allows you to move through life with a calmer spirit.

Proper exercise uses the idea that our bodies were designed to move and work, not sit behind a desk all day. Proper exercise is the gained when moving through the asanas, or yoga postures, which systematically work the entire body. While you may not have time to move through all the asanas in any given day, you should attempt to do them all in a one week period.

Proper breathing is the practice of breathing fully and regularly, using all of your lungs to increase the amount of oxygen breathed in. Yoga breathing exercises, or pranayama, teach how to maximize the breath in order to recharge the body and keep the mind calm and focused.

Proper diet is fairly obvious, but in a yoga framework, it means eating in moderation and only when hungry. Using food to fill a gap of loneliness or sadness will cause our senses to become dull so that we will not realize how much we ate or how it tasted. In yoga, food is used to sustain the body, not soothe the emotions.

The final principle of yoga, positive thinking and meditation, has a profound impact on our life by helping to remove the negative thoughts and allowing your mind to be calm and alert.

There are numerous benefits to practicing yoga.

- Stress relief: When you focus on breathing techniques, your body becomes calmer and your mind becomes quieter.

- Better mood: Your sense body confidence and well-being increases, and this directly correlates to lower blood pressure levels.

- Better sleep: Through your practice of yoga, you will learn to relax on command. Whether you take a class with a room full of strangers or use yoga DVD in your own home, you will be able to use the same relaxation techniques when you wish to fall asleep.

- Health: Moving your body and exercising is always a plus. Yoga poses increase flexibility and balance, strengthen muscles and help prevent aches and pains.

- Increased body awareness: Ordinarily speaking, people do not take the time to check in with their bodies and see how they are feeling. It's quite easy to ignore the small aches or problems we feel when we lead busy lives. At least until they turn into large issues. The practice of yoga encourages you to be mindful of your body and how it feels, even when you are not in a yoga studio.

- Learn what you need: Along the same idea as body awareness, you may notice that you don't feel as good as you thought you did. Your body will tell you if you need to take any corrective actions, like sitting up straighter, stretching more or taking a short walk because you have been sitting too long. Listen to your body and it will reward you by feeling better.

- Work faster: After you become a regular yoga practitioner, your mind will become centered, focused and clearer. You will find that your efficiency and productivity increase and your success rate will become higher.

- Combat minor illnesses: Studies have shown that yoga can help control headaches, stress, anxiety, asthma, and high blood pressure. The increased circulation any form of exercise provides will also stimulate your immune system.

- Concentration and creativity: When you are able to quiet your mind from meaningless distractions, you will be able to focus your thinking on problems at hand and find more creative solutions to them. You will develop a fresh outlook on life.

Misty Jordyn

CHAPTER TWO

YOGA AND BREATHING

Pranayama is the Sanskrit word for breathing. Proper breathing is one of the five principles of yoga and just practicing proper breathing can immediately enhance your life and health.

You can treat proper breathing as an exercise all on its own, without using any energy, and you can use it to completely relax yourself. From the yoga perspective, proper breathing provide more than oxygen to the blood, it is to control your essential life energy.

Our breath is sustenance for the body and the connection between our deepest resources and the universe at large. Connecting ourselves to the universe enhances our alertness and provide a fresh perspective on life.

Today people use deep breathing without any yoga context at all to control panic and anxiety attacks and to calm mental and emotional stress.

It is best to take time to practice proper breathing, it is the one thing that takes the least time to do yet it still has a large impact on our health. Too often in our modern life we breathe in short, fast, shallow breaths. Whether we are angry or stressed out or just too busy to pay attention, we do not take in sufficient oxygen, nor do we exhale enough carbon dioxide.

Without enough oxygen, we are not able to resist disease well and the health of our cells deteriorates. Lack of oxygen has recently been linked to cancer, heart disease and strokes. Make the time for a deep breathing ritual every morning and your health will improve.

There are days when there isn't even enough time for a 10 or 15 minute home yoga session. I encourage you to keep them to a minimum, but when you must, here are some breathing exercises you can do anywhere, at any time, to help keep your sense of inner peace and balance.

One great thing about deep breathing is that you can do it anywhere. I think the best time is while you are commuting to work. This time is generally not well spent and now you can make it a calming and healthful time.

Awareness of breath is an instant cue to your body to slow down and relax. Counting the breaths reduces stress and focuses the mind. The act of counting the breaths allows the body to breathe more deeply.

To begin mindful breathing, inhale deeply for a count of four. Hold for another count of four and finally exhale to a count of four. Try to fully expand your lungs while breathing in and fully empty your lungs as you exhale. In this manner you will fully oxygenate your blood and you will remove as many toxins as you can from your body. Try to fully deflate your lungs as you breathe out. This will help relax your shoulders and neck.

If you are not in your car, there are several stretches you can do to improve the oxygen content in your body. After a few minutes of breathing and stretching, you will be able to concentrate clearly on the tasks at hand, making this an excellent practice for the middle of the work day.

As you are doing your deep breathing exercises, pay attention to your surroundings. Focus on the beauty of nature and the sense of well-being your body is developing as you nourish your blood with oxygen.

While you should always try to perform at least a few yoga poses each day, there may be times when you can't. On those days it is absolutely critical that you take a few minutes from your hectic schedule and breathe deeply. You will return to your work invigorated, focused and ready to take on anything the universe throws at you.

CHAPTER THREE

STYLES OF YOGA

There are an incredible number of types of yoga available, each with its own individual emphasis and style. This list is not by any means exhaustive, but it will give you an idea the range of yoga styles available. With a little thought and planning, almost all of them can be modified to suit a busy lifestyle.

Ananda Yoga focuses on proper body alignment, controlled breathing and gentle postures that prepare the body for mediation.

Anusara Yoga was developed about 20 years ago and combines a playful spirit with challenging postures. Anusara is designed to help you connect with the divine in yourself and others.

Ashtanga Yoga is taught by Sri K. Pattabhi Jois. It combines synchronized breathing with a series of continuous postures that produce a purifying sweat that detoxifies both the muscles and organs. It is an athletic yoga and not suitable for beginners.

Bikram Yoga combines the traditional elements of fitness – muscular strength, endurance, cardiovascular health and weight loss. Bikram yoga is practiced in a hot room(95 to 105 degrees) to promote flexibility, injury prevention and greater detoxification.

Hatha Yoga is the basis of all yoga styles. It combines poses, breathing, mediation and kundalini into a system to achieve self-realization and enlightenment. Hatha Yoga is the most popular yoga style in the United States

Iyengar Yoga promotes flexibility, strength, balance and endurance by using poses that require precise alignment and coordinated breathing. Poses are held longer in Iyengar than in many other forms of yoga. Iyengar also uses props, such as blankets, cushions, blocks and straps to aid the less flexible in achieving the poses.

Jivamukti Yoga expresses the traditional ethical and spiritual aspects of yoga that are not always present in modern yoga. It is a vigorous form of yoga.

Kripalu Yoga is the yoga of consciousness. It is an introspective form of yoga that allows participants to hold poses while releasing spiritual and emotional blockages. Precise alignment is not as important as in other forms.

Kundalini Yoga focuses on awaking the energy at the base of the spine. Classes include poses, meditation, chanting and breathing exercises.

Power Yoga This is an American interpretation of Ashtanga yoga. Poses often resemble calisthenics and each pose flows directly into the next, providing a strong aerobic workout.

Sivananda Yoga This traditional style of yoga combines breathing, asanas, dietary restrictions, meditation and chanting.

Svaroopa Yoga This is considered a very approachable style for beginning students. Comfortable chair poses are often used. This form promotes transformation and healing.

Viniyoga This gentle, healing form of yoga is often used as therapy for individuals who are recuperating from surgery or have suffered injuries. It can be tailored to each person and can change as the person becomes stronger and more flexible.

Vinyasa Yoga This is a very active form of yoga that focuses on coordinating movement and breathwork.

White Lotus Yoga This is a modified Ashtanga yoga which combines meditation and breathwork.

Yin Yoga This is a yoga style that works more with the joints than the muscles. It focuses on working the connective tissues in the body. Most notable in this form of yoga is the long-held, passive nature of the postures. Don't be fooled into thinking it is an "easy" form, because the length of time to hold each pose can last up to twenty minutes.

CHAPTER FOUR

HOW DO I FIT YOGA
INTO MY BUSY DAY?

While spending an hour or more in your practice of yoga and meditation sounds wonderful, you can gain many benefits from a short routine as well. When you start using an abbreviated session, however, make sure you do it every day – you don't want to deprive yourself of the benefits of consistent practice.

Before you determine what kind of yoga can fit into your busy life, you need to examine your commitment to practicing yoga. Sit back and close your eyes. Consider all the reasons you want to do yoga, and then consider all the obstacles you will encounter to a regular yoga exercise schedule. If your reasons are shallow, for example, because you saw an attractive person entering a yoga studio, then now may not be the right time to begin. Your commitment level will be low and it will be too easy for you to stop.

If our commitment is strong, for example, to increase your health and sense of well-being, now is definitely the right time to begin. Your commitment level will be high and as you begin to feel the benefits of yoga your commitment will increase.

Are you ready to begin? Good.

There are several postures that can be done for short periods of time with great benefit. I suggest: crow squats, miracle bend or stretch pose. If you prefer, you can choose a series of poses and hold them for one minute each. A series of poses designed to clear the chakras would work well. One series that works well is this:

Tree Pose (Vrksasna)

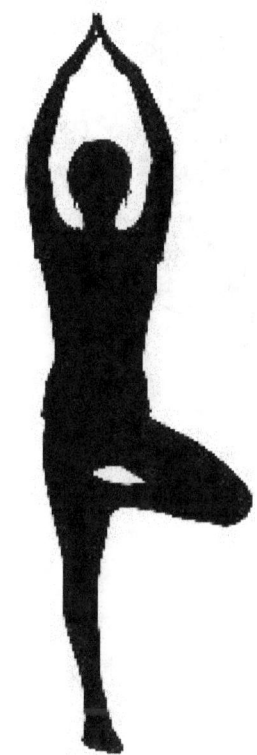

Goddess Pose (Deviasana)

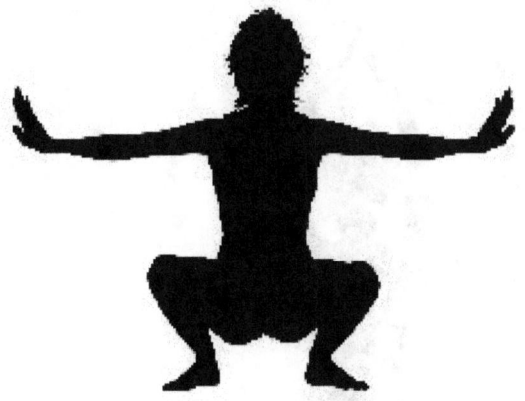

Boat Pose (Navasana)

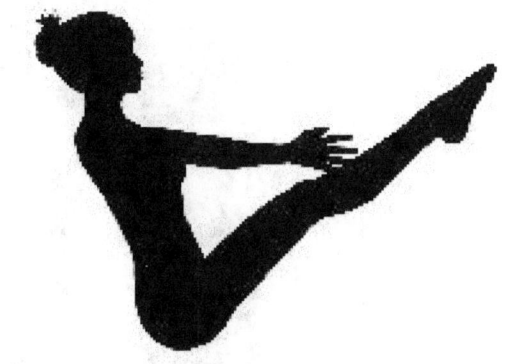

Camel Pose(Ustrasana)

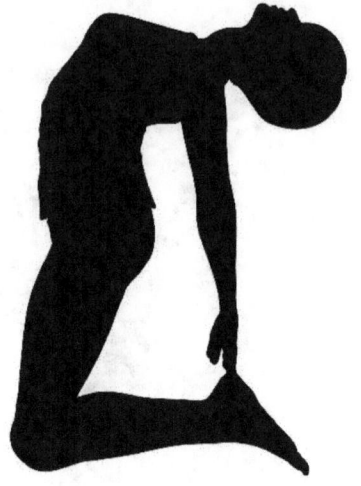

Supported Shoulder Stand (Salamba Sarvangasana)

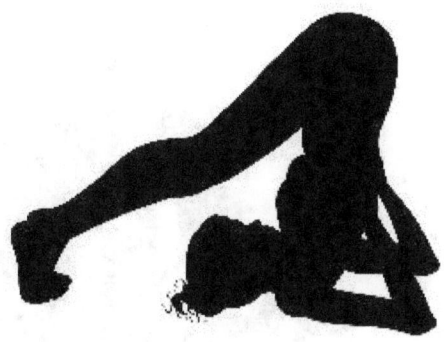

Easy Pose (Sukhasana)

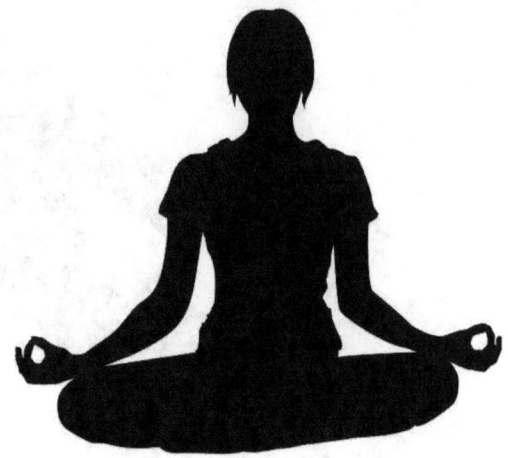

Corpse Pose (Savasna)

All that it implies. Lying on your back, palms up.

No matter which poses you choose to do, make sure to end with a few minutes of Corpse Pose to relax and allow your body and mind to return to the physical world.

Reciting a mantra is also a valuable way to clear the mind and focus the energy. You can choose a mantra that resonates with you and recite it for 11 minutes per day.

Here are five powerful Sanskrit mantras and their meanings.

1. OM Om represents the cycle of life from birth to death and then back to re-birth. It is the original sound of the universe and has no translation.

2. Om Namah Shivaya "I bow to Shiva." A modern translation of this mantra is "I honor the divinity within myself." This mantra can be used to develop self-confidence because it reminds us that we are made of divine energy and should treat ourselves with the reverence this requires.

3. Lokah Smastah Sukhino Bhavantu "May all beings be free and happy and may my own life contribute to the freedom and happiness for all." This lovely sentiment will aid you to live a life of peace and being of service to the greater good.

4. Om Saha Naavavatu, Saha Nau Bunaktu, Saha Veeryam Karavaavahai, Tejasvi Aavadheetamatsu Maa

Vidvishaavahai Om "May the Lord protect and bless us. May he nourish us and strengthen us to work together for the good of all humanity. May our learning be brilliant and purposeful. May we never turn against one another." This is a wonderful mantra to use at beginnings – the start of a yoga class, the beginning of the day or even when opening a new business. This mantra unites all who say it in a sphere of unity and cooperation.

5. Om Gum Ganapatayei Namah I bow to Ganesh who can remove all obstacles. I pray for blessings and protection." Ganesh is the god of wisdom and success. He is also the destroyer of obstacles. This is an excellent mantra for challenging times in life, and also while traveling.

To truly get into the habit of yoga, daily practice is essential. It takes 30 days to change a habit and 90 days to confirm a habit. In 120 days the new habit is a part of you and in 1000 days you have mastered the new habit. This is amazing to me. 1000 days is 2 years and 9 months (give or take a couple of days). 2 years and 9 months to mastery.

Misty Jordyn

CHAPTER FIVE

YOGA IN THE TWENTY FIRST CENTURY

Yoga has benefitted for advanced technology in that there are many smartphone apps to help you start and maintain your yoga practice. The following list of apps are available for free or a small fee. These are not even close to the number of apps you can find, but this is a representative selection that lets you see what is available for you.

Check them out and see which will support you in your goal of regular yoga practice.

Yoga Studio

Yoga Studio comes with 65 premade video yoga and meditation sessions that range from ten to sixty minutes. You may create your own class with their library of poses and 'pose blocks', which are poses that are normally grouped together. The ambient sounds and music may be changed to your liking and you can automatically set a reminder in your calendar so you don't forget to practice yoga every day.

Yoga Studio is available at the iTunes store for $3.99. It is not currently available for Android devices.

Yoga.com Studio

Yoga.com Studio has many programs and poses that are planned for all yoga practitioners, from beginner to advanced levels. It comes with a video library of preset programs and poses. You can make your own program or just add individual poses. There is a built-in community for you to share your work or search for other people's custom programs. Like Yoga Studio, it has a schedule feature.

Yoga.com Studio is free on Android and $3.00 at the iTunes store.

Daily Yoga

Daily Yoga has a video library of over 50 yoga classes and over 400 workout poses, with background music. Beginners will find seven yoga plans add a variety of intensities, exercises and durations. For the more advanced modules, you will need a subscription to Daily Yoga.

Daily Yoga is free on both Android and at the iTunes Store.

Pocket Yoga

Pocket Yoga allows you to practice at your own pace and time. It's like a yoga studio in your pocket because it has detailed audio and visual instructions for many different poses. Each exercise is accompanied by full text write-ups of benefits of the exercise and instructions for forming the pose correctly. There are three different practices, durations and difficulty levels. The app keeps track of your most used combinations for future reference.

Pocket Yoga is available at the iTunes store and on Android for $2.99.

Pocket Yoga Practice Builder

The Pocket Yoga Practice Builder is built from the Pocket Yoga app. Designed for serious yoga students and teachers, it allows them to create and save their individual routines and classes. There is a library of over 200 poses that can be scheduled for the order and time required. The app also recommends combinations of poses based on established yoga practices. Once you have designed your routine, you can save them and then share via email, AirDrop or you can download them as PDF documents.

Pocket Yoga Practice Builder can be found at the iTunes store for $6.99. It is not currently available for Android.

5 Minute Yoga

5 Minute Yoga contains 350 short, effective yoga classes that can be completed in about five minutes – perfect for our fast-paced lives. The sessions are taken from a large library of poses and instructions. Each session has a timer to make sure you hold the pose for the appropriate length of time. There is also a music library.

5 Minute Yoga is available at the iTunes store for 99 cents. It is not currently available for Android.

Another way to incorporate yoga into your modern life is to subscribe to an online service that will deliver a yoga session to you every day, or find one of the many yoga websites that will guide you through a session whenever you are ready.

Misty Jordyn

CHAPTER SIX

YOGA WHILE TRAVELING

Mixing yoga while traveling can be difficult, particularly if you are traveling for work and your time is not your own. Your schedule is thrown off, you may not sleep as well and if you have a very small hotel room, you may not have space for many poses.

It is easy to tell yourself that you will exercise while away from home, but it doesn't always work out that way. Traveling tends to take up all your time, and then some. There are so many things to do, old friends to visit, new friends to make, work demands that must be met and of course the physical process of getting from one place to the other always seems to take longer than anticipated.

Despite the craziness of travel, you should strive to set some time aside for yourself every day. The best times are either first thing in the morning or last thing in the evening. Take these moments to breathe deeply, flow through some simple poses and reconnect with yourself and the universe. Make the time and you will feel better about yourself.

Below are some tips to keep yourself on track while you're away.

Be Prepared

Bring your mat and yoga clothes with you. You can purchase a small travel mat from Manduka that easily fits in your luggage.

Set Goals and Make a Commitment

You cannot reach a goal if you haven't set it. Think about your upcoming trip and realistically (that's the key here) think about when you will have time for yoga. Consider when you prefer to practice yoga and what you are currently working on. Commit to yourself that you will continue to work on these goals.

Be Consistent

No matter where you are or how experienced you are, it pays to remain consistent in your practice, both at home and away. When you set your goals and make your commitment, set a specific time to devote to yoga, proper breathing and meditation. If you cannot practice every day that you are away, commit to the number of days you will practice.

Anything is Better than Nothing

It is better to start than not start. Reaching some of our goals is by far preferable than not reaching any of them. If you are new to yoga or new to exercise while traveling, it may take a few trips out of town to get used to the added discipline it will take to exercise while away. Do your best and be proud of yourself.

Find New Places

Find new and beautiful places to inspire your practice of yoga. The front desk of your hotel can tell you if they hold yoga classes in the hotel. The pool, rooftop or balcony may offer beautiful scenery for meditation. You can also, if you have time, explore the parks and public spaces of the city you are in.

CHAPTER SEVEN

YOGA FOR STRESS AND ANXIETY

Yoga is a great stress reliever and it can also help relieve the symptoms of anxiety, which is often found hand in hand with stress. When we focus our attention to our bodies and breathing, yoga helps keep anxiety at bay while releasing the physical manifestations of the tension we feel.

Anxiety is the most prevalent mental illness in the United States and it affects almost 40 million adults, which is 18 % of the nation's adults. 20 % of teens also suffer from anxiety, so it looks as though this trend isn't going to change for a long time.

The following yoga poses can be done individually, in this order or you could even just pick and choose a few that make you feel better. With the exception of the headstand, these poses are designed with beginners in mind. If you are a more advanced yogi or yogini, you can add in some balancing poses like Eagle Pose,

Tree Pose and Half Moon Pose. Try to hold each standing pose for between 30 and 60 seconds on each side.

Focus on your breath as you work your way through the poses. You can close your eyes to help you focus on your pose, go within and achieve a more meditative state. The goal here is to do whatever helps you alleviate your stress and anxiety. These poses alleviate stress and anxiety by forcing us to focus on the present moment and not whatever our monkey mind has in store for us.

If you are new to yoga, practicing restorative yoga (also called active relaxation) is a wonderful way to begin. Restorative yoga places emphasis on stillness, relaxation and a calmer state of mind. It uses props, including blocks, bolsters, blankets and straps to help support and align the body and allow it to settle into the pose as best as it can. Using these props allows the beginning yogi and yogini to hold poses longer than they would be able to.

Above all, remember that yoga is a practice and not a competition. Begin where you are comfortable and advance with slow caution. Listen to your body, don't push beyond what feels good and you will be able to avoid injury.

Anjali Mudra (Salutation Seal)

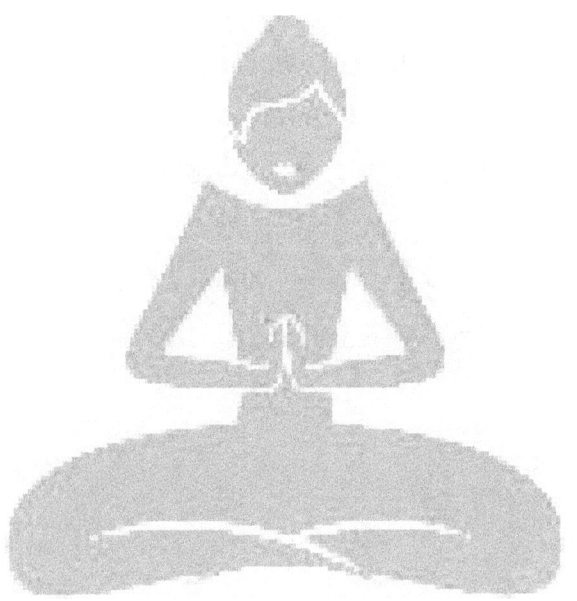

The Anjali Mudra induces a state of meditative awareness. It is commonly performed with hands in the center of the heart chakra, which represents the balance and harmony between our left and right sides that are united at our center. This balance is physical, emotional and mental and when we begin our yoga session, we go to our center in preparation for meditation and contemplation. It is best to start this pose while seated in a comfortable cross-legged position with our eyes closed.

Sukhasana (Easy Pose)

'Pictured Above'

The Easy Pose has both physical and emotional benefits which help amplify your serenity and tranquility, eliminate anxiety and relieve both physical and mental exhaustion. It promotes inner calm and a sense of groundedness as well as opening your hips and lengthening your spine. When in this pose, focus on your breath and sit still with a straight spine for at least 60 seconds.

Marjaryasana (Cat Pose)

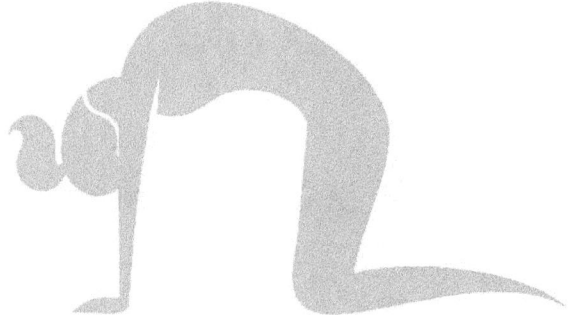

This pose gives the spine and internal organs a gentle massage while relieving stress. It is often paired with the Cow Pose as the practitioner is inhaling for a simple, gentle vinyasa. Cat Pose stimulates the digestive tract and is good for overall health. Proper alignment is when the wrists are directly under the shoulders and the knees are directly under the hips.

Bitilasana (Cow Pose)

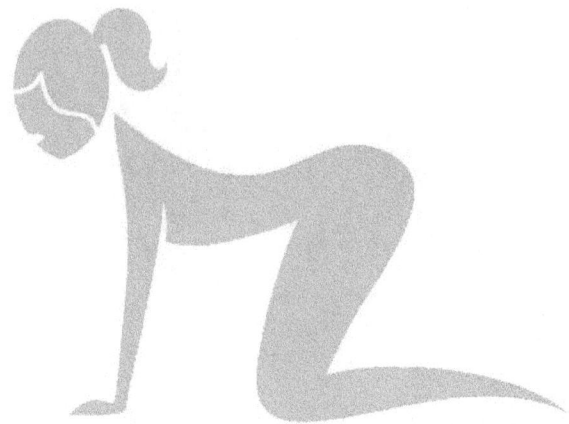

Cow Pose is a gentle, easy way to warm up and stretch the spine. As noted above, it is often alternated with Cat Pose. This pose calms the mind, relieves stress, promotes emotional balance and helps to stimulate the kidneys and adrenal glands. Wrist and knee positions are the same as Cat Pose, wrists under the shoulders and knees under the hips.

Uttana Shishosana (Extended Puppy Pose)

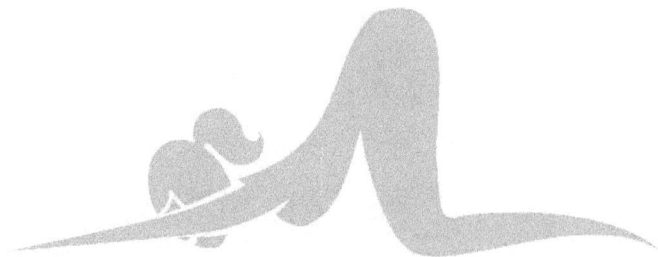

This pose lengthens the spine, calms the mind and invigorates the body. It looks like a cross between Downward Facing Dog and Child's Pose. This pose can also relieve some of the symptoms of chronic stress, insomnia and tension.

Paschimottanasana (Seated Forward Bend)

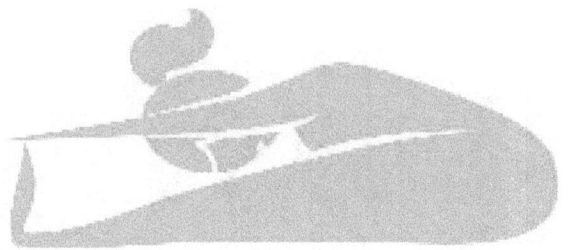

Seated Forward Bend will help your distracted mind unwind and regain its focus. This is a basic pose, but don't think it isn't challenging. In addition to relieving stress and anxiety, it stretches the hamstrings, lower back and spine, relieves the symptoms of PMS and menopause, improves digestion, stimulates organs including the liver, ovaries, kidneys and uterus, and reduces fatigue. When in this position, keep your feet flexed and lower your forehead to your knees.

Janu Sirsasana (Head-to-Knee Forward Bend)

This pose is a forward bend suitable for all levels of yoga students. This pose also incorporates a spinal twist. You can settle into this pose with both arms reaching for your extended food or by rotating sideways and extending your arm over your head. This pose has a variety of benefits, including: calming the brain, relieving mild anxiety, fatigue, menstrual discomfort, headache, and insomnia.

Salamba Sirsasana (Supported Headstand)

Please note that if you have glaucoma or high blood pressure you should not do inverted asanas. If you are pregnant, inverted asanas are not safe once your center of balance has shifted from normal.

Headstands, done with the proper alignment, calm the brain and strengthen the body. Anxiety is eased when the blood flow is reversed and you focus your breath and body on the present moment. Your heart is also given a bit of a rest because it is not pumping blood back up from your lower body.

If you are a beginner, it is good to practice this pose against a wall for stability.

Your weight should be resting on your forearms and shoulders, not your head and neck. There should be enough space between your head and the mat for a piece of paper to slip between them.

Eka Pada Rajakapotasana (Half-Pigeon Pose)

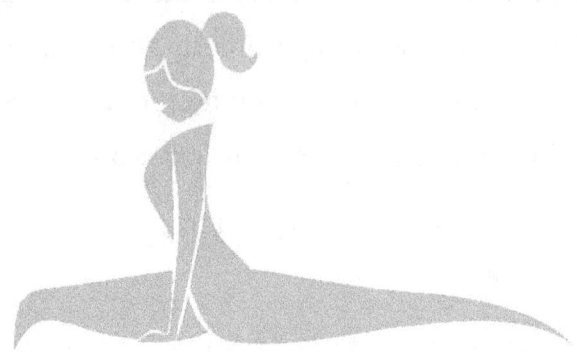

Start on all fours and slide your right knee forward toward your right hand. Lower your right hip onto a bolster, pillow, or folded blanket as you extend your left leg back, toes pointed. Remain upright using hands to support you, or lower down to forearms. Breathe into the pose as you inch your right shin closer to the mat. Carefully come up to downward-facing dog, then lower onto your left hip to repeat on other side.

Setu Bandha Sarvangasana (Supported Bridge Pose)

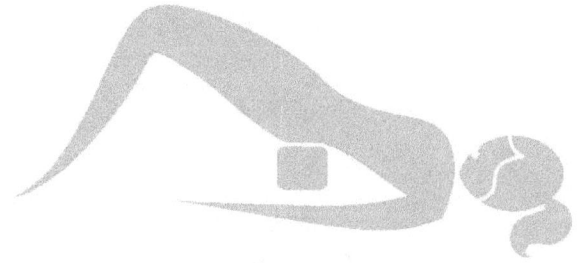

Lie on your back with your knees bent, feet planted flat on the floor, hip-distance apart. Extend your arms by your sides and roll your shoulder blades in toward one another to feel a slight lift in the chest. Carefully lift your hips off the ground and slide a yoga block directly under your sacrum, the large, triangular bone at the base of your spine. (Note: Always come into bridge pose before you place the block under your sacrum—don't try to lie directly on the block.)

As you rest here, arms can remain by your sides, stretched overhead, or straight out in a T-shape. Beginners can keep the block at its lowest height, then rotate it for a higher lift. To come out of the pose, press down into your feet and lift your hips. Remove the block and gently lower back to the floor.

Balasana (Child's Pose)

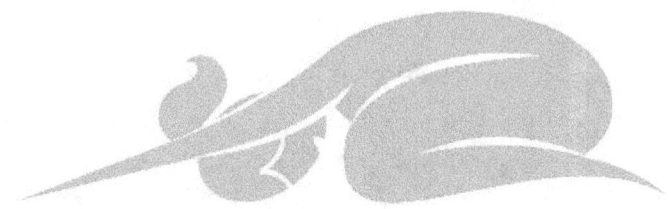

Child's Pose is a perfect follow up to Supported Headstand. Start by sitting on your knees and bending forward with your arms outstretched or by your side. When you place your forehead on the ground, you will relieve more physical stress and emotional anxiety. This is a good pose to do between any two more challenging asanas. If you prefer, you can put your arms alongside your body instead of over your head – the only rule is to do what feels best for you.

Savasana (Corpse Pose)

Although it looks simple, Savasna is one of the most challenging asanas. Savasna is truly achieved when the body and mind are totally relaxed – that's the challenge. This pose allows the body's nervous system to integrate everything gained from the day's yoga practice before going back to the stresses of 'normal life.' While laying on your back, allow your body to melt as deeply into the mat as possible with each breath. This pose requires a minimum of five minutes to complete.

Misty Jordyn

CHAPTER EIGHT

YOGA FOR INSOMNIA

Almost everyone has a sleepless night once in a great while. Whether you are overburdened at work and can't seem to 'shut it off' at home, are having problems with some personal relationships or even if you're too excited about wonderful things going on in your life, you may wind up missing a night of sleep.

Missing one night of sleep is not so bad, but when your sleeplessness drags on for two, three, or even more nights in a row, it's time to address the problem before it becomes a chronic condition.

Not everyone requires the same amount of sleep. The generally accepted healthy ranges of sleep are between seven and nine hours per night. You may need more or less than that range – the only person who knows how much sleep you need is you.

If you have insomnia, it's not bad enough that you didn't get enough (or any!) rest the night before, but the next day you need to deal with some pretty difficult symptoms, including: debilitating sleepiness, irritability, anxiety, depression, headache, digestive issues and trouble maintaining your attention. Insomnia can lead to dangerous levels of sleepiness or lack of mental focus and has been linked to car accidents, medical errors and even chronic diseases like depression, anxiety, high blood pressure, obesity and even cancer.

Topping the list of causes of insomnia is stress, then anxiety and depression. There are other causes of insomnia, including medications (both prescription and over the counter), caffeine, nicotine, alcohol, changes in work or home schedule, medical conditions (difficulty breathing, chronic pain or frequent urination), poor sleep habits, and eating too much too late in the day. You can also suffer from insomnia because you worry too much about not being able to fall asleep.

The rate people develop or suffer from insomnia increases as they age because they change their sleep patterns, decrease their energy levels, their health tends to decline, and they tend to increase the strength and number of medications they are on.

Research indicates that yoga can help. We already know that helps combat the symptoms of stress, anxiety and depression –

many of these are felt by people as they become older. Another study has shown that yoga also helps the brain avoid cognitive arousal. This name is a bit misleading. Cognitive arousal isn't when your brain is thinking, it is when your brain is racing when you are trying to or have just fallen asleep.

Evening yoga practice has also decreased insomnia in menopausal women.

It is better to use yoga to combat your insomnia first thing in the morning. It is more helpful to do a vigorous yoga practice, or as vigorous as you can manage, in the morning. This will help your body and your hormone levels support a better night's sleep. Even if you are very tired, a gentle practice will help get you moving and loosen up the tension that your body is carrying after a night of insomnia.

After your morning practice, it is important to pay attention to what you eat and drink throughout the day, because they can affect how you sleep in the evening. Consuming caffeine, alcohol, stimulating medication or drugs will keep you from sleeping well in the evening. Smoking cigarettes will also keep you up later at night and will destroy your health.

If you are able, spending 15 minutes outside, in nature (or as close to nature as you can get) will help you reconnect to a quieter, more peaceful life.

Once you get home from work or school, having an earlier dinner and then, after an hour for digestion, a gentle yoga practice will prepare your mind and body for relaxation and sleep. Use poses that you personally find relaxing and quieting and incorporate breathing processes that are calming as well. A guided visualization or meditation will help calm your nervous system and prepare it for sleeping. Evening screen time should end an hour before you go to bed, and at least while you are suffering from insomnia, reading thrilling books before bed should be stopped.

As your yoga practice continues you can place yourself in a state of yoga nidra. Yoga nidra means 'yogic sleep' and is more like a trance. It is a state between wakefulness and sleep, called the hypnogogic state. It is easiest to reach this state in the Savasana pose (described below). Yoga nidra can last about 20 minutes and you won't feel yourself slipping into it, you will only realize you have reached it when you wake from it. Once you arouse from your yoga nidra state, it will be much easier to fall asleep for the night.

If you still have problems falling asleep or if you continue to wake in the middle of the night and cannot fall asleep, try breathing exercises or do the yoga poses listed in the next section.

Practicing yoga in a bed is generally discouraged because you may fall asleep, breaking your meditation. Because your ultimate goal is to fall asleep, yoga in bed is perfectly acceptable.

To perform Savasana for sleep, follow these steps:

- Lie flat on your back with your arms at your sides and your palms facing upward. Your legs should be slightly parted and your eyes should be closed.

- Focus on your right arm. With your eyes closed, visualize the arm in your mind's eye, feeling all the sensations in your skin, muscles and bones in that arm. Feel the blood flowing through your veins.

- Inhale and make a fist with your right hand, lifting your arm from the floor or bed. Hold it up for a moment, then drop it while exhaling. Relax the arm and let it lie still.

- Follow this routine for your left arm, right leg, left leg and then torso. Tense and relax every part of your body in this order. When you have finished, your whole body should feel relaxed. Focus on the bed (or floor) beneath you and how your body makes contact with it. Visualize yourself melting completely into the floor, surrendering your body to gravity. Finally, empty your mind of any distracting thoughts.

It may take more than one or two nights for this pose to help you fall asleep, so be persistent. Even if it doesn't help immediately, enjoy the relaxation and calmness your mind feels while in this pose.

CHAPTER NINE

YOGA IN YOUR BED

The next time you are lying awake in bed, don't count sheep or become frustrated, grab your yoga mat instead. The relaxation yoga provides can help combat insomnia and help you get a deep, restful night's sleep. Just closing your eyes and taking deep, slow breaths can calm the body and mind.

Before you begin your yoga for insomnia practice, put your pajamas on, brush your teeth and do everything you need to prepare for sleeping. That way, once you are done, you can take your relaxed, calm body straight to sleep. And hey, if you fall asleep during Corpse Pose, that's fine, too. Each of these poses can be done in bed, so you won't need to even get up, unless your partner is already sleeping.

Viparita Karani (Upside-Down Relaxation)

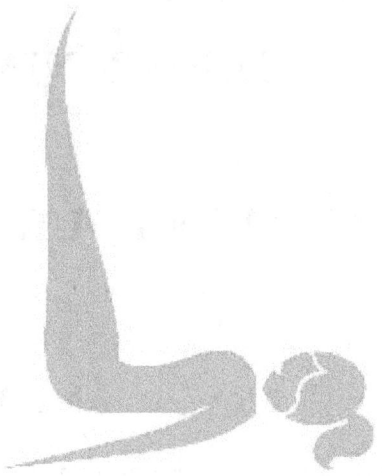

Form an L with your body by putting your legs against the wall or your headboard and scooching your behind up to the wall. Move your arms above your head and rest them on the bed. If this is uncomfortable for you, cross your arms over your chest. Inhale and exhale slowly for several minutes. If you have been walking, wearing high heels or otherwise on your feet all day, this will reward your feet with some restorative relaxation.

Supta Baddha Konasana (Modified Goddess)

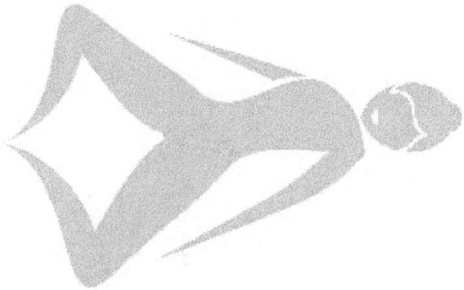

Move from Upside Dow Relaxation to your 'normal' lying on your back sleeping pose. Bring the soles of your feet together and let your knees and legs fall to each side, creating a diamond shape. Raise your arms over your head and rest them on the bed above your head. If your head or shoulders feel any tension, place a pillow under them. Lengthen your neck and allow it to relax. Slightly lift your pelvis off the bed for a moment, straightening your lower back. Hold this pose for 12 breaths.

Supta Jaṭhara Parivartānāsana (Spinal Twist)

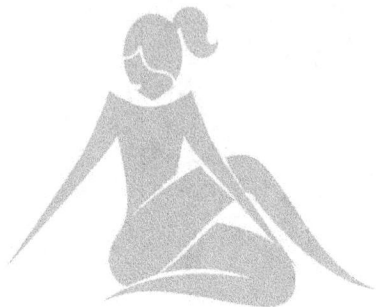

Straighten your legs and stretch your arms to each side, keeping your palms up. Bend your right knee until your foot is flat on the mattress and up close to your behind. Slowly lower your right knee across your body and use your left hand to provide gentle pressure on top of the thigh. Turn your head toward your left hand and hold for 10 to 12 breaths. Repeat on the other side.

Savasana (Corpse Pose)

Lay on your back and allow your body and mind to fully relax. With each breath in, feel more muscles relax and with each breath out, sink deeper into your bed.

Misty Jordyn

CHAPTER TEN

CURING A HEADACHE OR BACK ACHE WITH YOGA

Modern life is often lived at a headlong rush, at the expense of being mindful of our bodies. We carry tension throughout our bodies and this leads to headaches, backaches, tension and stress. Because we are too busy and stressed to be mindful, we shut out the minor aches and pains we feel and just press on, ignoring the messages our bodies are sending.

Headaches are the bane of the modern world. Often, people move throughout their day feeling "off", or unhappy or angry and not really realizing why. One of the reasons is that they have a headache but have tried to shut out the pain and keep powering through their day.

While taking a pain reliever can seem like the right thing to do, there are other, more natural ways to relieve your pain that don't involve putting chemicals into your body. *Viparita Karani (Upside-Down Relaxation)* for five to ten minutes will stretch the muscles of your neck and help you relax. The instructions for this pose are in the previous chapter. Once your legs are up on the wall, place your hands on the mat above your head or rest them on your belly. Close your eyes, relax your jaw and drop your chin. Breathe in deeply and slowly, releasing the tension from your body.

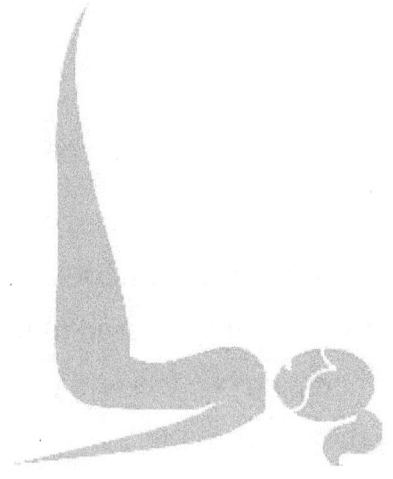

Viparita Karani (Upside-Down Relaxation)

Back pain is practically epidemic in the United States. It's no wonder, as we spend too much time sitting, have poor posture and many of us carry around extra weight that our spines and core muscles must compensate for.

If it is your back that is giving you trouble, *Supta Jaṭhara Parivartānāsana (Spinal Twist)* will give you relief and help prevent future pain by strengthening the muscles and ligaments near your spine. The instructions for this pose are found in the previous chapter. Please be very careful when beginning this pose. Move slowly, deliberately and carefully into and throughout the pose. Stop before anything begins to hurt or feel pulled. It is better to stretch a bit every day and work into the full pose than to go too fast and possibly make your back hurt more.

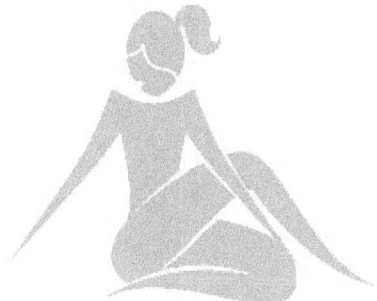

Supta Jaṭhara Parivartānāsana (Spinal Twist)

Misty Jordyn

CHAPTER ELEVEN

YOGA FOR KIDS

Growing up in the world today can be difficult for kids of all ages. Children are exposed to more news at an earlier age and worry about terrorism, climate change, terrorism and politics – none of which they can affect in any way. They also worry about issues closer to home: bullies, grades, divorcing parents, friends, dating – the list goes on and on. It's no wonder they feel stress.

It can be difficult to know how to help our kids when they are feeling stress. Our first inclination is to step in and solve the problem for them, but this isn't going to help them in the long run. What we need to do is provide them with the tools to solve their own problems, and one of the biggest hurdles children must leap on their path to adulthood is behaving mindfully rather than reacting to everything that happens immediately.

The earlier in life a person begins their practice of yoga, the better off they will be. It is important, however, to make sure that yoga isn't just one more thing to squeeze into an already overscheduled day.

The many benefits of yoga for children

Yoga teaches physical skills like strength, flexibility, stamina, coordination and balance, but it is not the only exercise that can do that. Unlike gymnastics, dance or team sports, yoga is non-competitive and allows adults and children alike to focus on his or her own progress. In fact, it may be the only area in a child's life where there is no competition, grading of judgment. Team sports are said to promote self-discipline and confidence, but yoga does this as well, while promoting creativity, compassion and self-expression.

All parents are concerned with their children's physical fitness and health and want them to be active, but the price of team sports can be too high – sports related injuries and concussions are becoming more common in younger children and this damage can follow them through their lives. Yoga teaches proper body alignment and promotes flexibility, helping kids use their bodies safely.

Children need a practice that suits their emotional and physical needs and a course or video designed for young children is a good place to start.

Yoga and ADD

Kids who have ADD or ADHD can benefit from yoga. Yoga's calming, relaxing breathing techniques and concentrated focus on specific postures helps calm children and move them in a positive direction.

A 2004 study in the *Journal of Attention Disorders* reported that boys of age 8 to 13 who practiced yoga once a week for five months had increased concentration, and both physical and mental discipline. They also showed improved confidence. Their parents reported that the boys were less hyperactive. This study stopped short of concluding that yoga could be used in lieu of medication.

Fun poses to try with your kids

If you are the DIY type, you can do some easy poses with your children. All you need is a space to spread out and a spirit of fun. Children love to imagine themselves as different animals or other objects, so use that to your benefit and make noises, use music or even make up stories to go with the poses.

Don't take yoga too seriously with your kids. Kids love running, jumping, playing and goofing around, so let them be themselves when they're practicing yoga.

For example, it's okay to laugh at how silly you look with your bottoms high up in the air in Downward Facing Dog. When you child successfully completes a complicated asana, give them a high five. Don't worry if they don't want to meditate right away, or if they even just start laughing when you do.

Yoga is a practice, a process that continues, hopefully, throughout life.

Tree Pose with a Partner

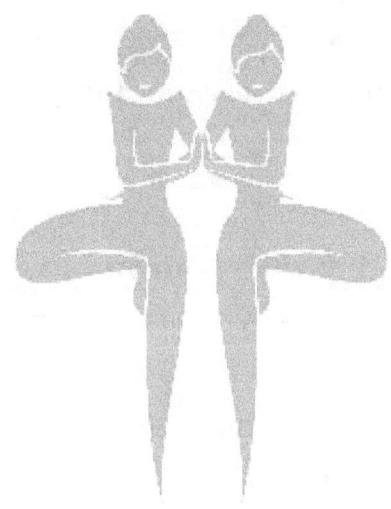

This pose teaches support for others coordination and balance. Stand hip to hip next to your partner, both facing the same way. Imagine yourself as a strong, tall tree in the forest. Your feet are the roots of the tree so stand very tall with your feet together. Place your arm around your partner's back and focus on an unmoving point on the wall. Life one foot off the ground while transferring your weight to the other leg. Press your lifted foot into the calf or thigh of your standing leg, keeping your knee pointed outward. Help stabilize each other and lift your free hand to join your partner's, over your heads. Imagine the wobbliness you feel is the wind moving through your branches. Lean into each other while standing tall. Find the strength in you and your partner and how you work together.

Downward Facing Dog

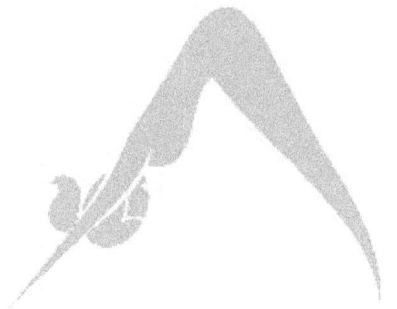

Downward facing dog stretches the back and strengthens the arms and legs. This pose mimics a dog stretching when he wakes up in the morning. Get down on your hands and knees like a puppy, with your knees and hands hip and shoulder width apart. Spread your fingers out and press them into the floor. Take a deep breath in and arch your back. Curl your toes under, exhale and straighten your legs, pushing yourself up into an inverted V. When you are in the pose, you can bark or growl like a dog for fun.

And as always, it is good to end with Savasna.

CHAPTER TWELVE

YOGA AND TEENS

If you think young children are under stress, teens have it much worse. Not only do they have the competition and daily judgment younger children have, by the time they get to high school they are playing for huge stakes. College scholarships, exclusive admissions into top programs and competitive sports that can make or break a student's career long after high school are just some of the worries they have. There's also the physiological, emotional and social aspects of their lives that are unlike any other time they will ever live through.

Every teen has been born after 9/11. The country has been in many wars, the world has suffered through natural disasters, a nuclear plant disaster, and poverty and hunger are on the rise throughout the world.

It's no wonder they're under stress and can turn to unhealthy habits to cope.

Many teens are able to cope with these stresses, but it is good to encourage healthy relaxation for your teens as a practice they can take through their adult lives.

The most challenging part of bringing teens to yoga is the initial presentation. Teens need to know how spending their valuable time on yoga will help them and be worth their time. Teens think they are the center of the universe and know that everyone is watching them. Using their natural egocentricity is the way to get them interested. Begin with a question – let them talk about who they are and why they are in the class. If that won't work, ask them to share one activity they truly enjoy.

After the introductions, use every bit of information they give you as a catalyst for your class. Use their interests in your examples, find players, teams or other examples of their heroes who use yoga in their lives.

Make sure they know why the hard work of some of the advanced poses matters. They will persevere if they know their investment will yield focus for good grades or strength for their games. Ask what is in it for them and remind them often.

Teens can move through poses fairly quickly and they want to. They don't want to hear about every nuance of each pose, so cover the basics and keep them moving. Build in the details a little bit at a time. They will want to focus on breathing and safety to get their benefits.

Work with the teens as equal partners. Ask them guiding questions, like 'How do you cope with a situation when you feel insecure?' Listening to them respectfully will yield their own wisdom and depth of feeling that will amaze you.

Teens often want to just relax, but there is not time for relaxation in their day. Yoga time can be that relaxation time. Even if students only spend their time focusing their mind on their breath and consciously relaxing. This conscious relaxation is completely different from the usual video games/internet surfing/social media relaxation and will leave their minds and bodies in a better place. The problem with the relaxation feelings from these screen-based activities is that teens don't know how to recreate these feelings outside of screen time.

Yoga, on the other hand, creates a clear awareness of a person's state of being and helps them develop the skills to shift back to that state when necessary. This also helps facilitate emotional intelligence by having teens listen to their own inner voice that can be drowned out due to the fear and anxiety they often feel.

Even just conscious breathing can help students cope with stress.

Teens struggle with issues of control and power. They have more responsibilities and power than ever before, but they still have to live within what seem to be arbitrary boundaries set by teachers and parents. Their breath, however, is something they can absolutely control. Five minutes of intentional breathing can be a powerful way to prepare for a test, interview, performance or even just a school day.

Teens are quick to point out that we are always breathing, so we must be doing it right. Explaining to them how breathing, particularly intentional breathing works, helps them realize there is a lot to learn about breathing past the involuntary muscle movements.

Finally, breathing changes the energy in the body from stress to relaxation. Most teens want to be able to take their stress and turn it into relaxation, so you should be able to keep their attention with this.

Some good poses to begin with include:

Brahmari (Bee Buzzing Breath)

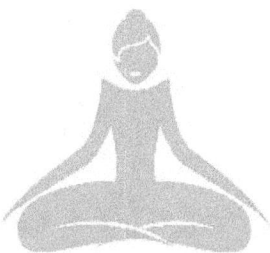

Bee Buzzing Breath can be done in any position, but ideally sitting up straight with a lifted chest and eyes closed. Begin by taking a deep breath in and then humming out when exhaling. Relax and observe the effects before repeating. Although it sounds funny, you can't do this seriously without feeling calmer. The sounds you are making take your attention from your brain and into your voice and heart, giving you a mental break. Long exhales are also very calming for the nervous system.

Garudasana (Eagle Pose)

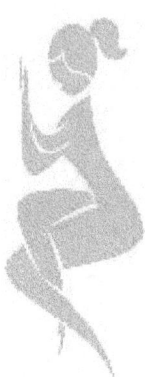

This pose can be done seated or standing. Begin with steadying your gaze on one spot and engage your arms and legs in the positon an eagle takes. This takes the energy of your brain and puts it into your body. Imagine yourself soaring over the landscape as your mental pressure releases and you begin to feel steady and clear.

Marjaryasana (Cat Pose) and Bitilasana (Cow Pose)

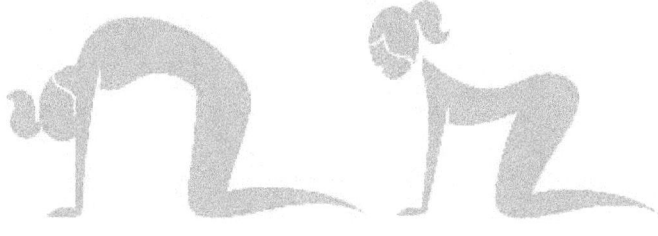

Flowing between these two poses releases mental tension, loosens the spine and leaves the body refreshed and renewed.

Uttanasana (Seated or Standing Forward Bend)

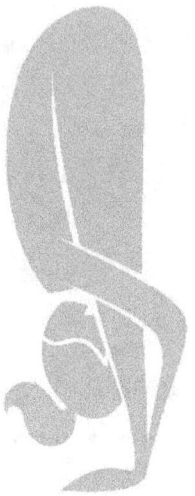

Bend forward and let your head and arms hang. Blood will flow to your head and this extra circulation is rejuvenating and refreshing. You can also support your head on a chair. This will cool your brain while supporting your head.

Balasana (Child's Pose)

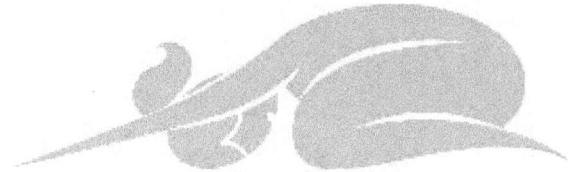

Child's Pose redirects the focus inward and can help dispel any feelings of stress. It evokes a sense of safety and comfort, and allows for a time of total relaxation.

Adho Mukha Savanasana (Downward Dog)

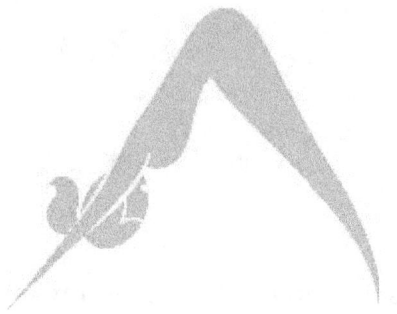

Downward facing dog stretches the back and strengthens the arms and legs. This pose mimics a dog stretching when he wakes up in the morning. Get down on your hands and knees like a puppy, with your knees and hands hip and shoulder width apart. Spread your fingers out and press them into the floor. Take a deep breath in and arch your back. Curl your toes under, exhale and straighten your legs, pushing yourself up into an inverted V. When you are in the pose, you can bark or growl like a dog for fun.

CHAPTER THIRTEEN

THE MEDITATIVE STATE

When a person meditates, the body undergoes a series of physical changes that reduce stress and depression. This chapter lists many studies and results that link meditation to greater emotional, mental and physical health.

On the physical level, meditation has the following effects:

- Lowers blood pressure to a more normal level

- Decreases tension-related pain including headache, muscle tightness and ulcers

- Lessens insomnia

- Lowers the level of lactic acid in the blood which reduces physical anxiety

- Increases serotonin, which improves mood

- Strengthens the immune system

- Increases energy

On the mental level, meditation allows the brain to use an alpha brainwave pattern, allowing relaxation and healing. The effects include:

- Decreased anxiety

- Increased emotional stability

- Increased happiness

- Increased creativity

- Clarity

- Peace of mind

- Problems appear more manageable

- Sharpens thought

The Emotional Benefits of Meditation

There is no disputing the fact that meditation provides strong, long-lasting benefits for the mental and emotional states of its practitioners. The regular practice of meditation enhances a positive outlook on life and a positive self-image.

Meditation Reduces General Anxiety and Stress

Open Monitoring Meditation, the practice of being aware of thoughts without acting on them, reduces the density of grey matter in the stress and anxiety related areas of the brain. Participants in a study from the University of Wisconsin-Madison reported an increased ability to focus on their current surroundings without becoming upset over any particular thing. The ability to allow things to pass without strong reaction reduces anxiety and stress.

Meditation Reduces Symptoms of Panic Disorder

A paper in the American Journal of Psychiatry reported that after three months of meditation training, 20 of 22 patients showed substantial decreases in the effects of panic and anxiety. When followed up at a later date, those benefits were still being felt.

Meditation Increases Brain Growth

Harvard neuroscientists studied 16 people during and after an 8 week mindfulness course. Participants used guided meditation and incorporated mindfulness throughout their daily activities. At the end of the study, MRI scans showed an increase in the gray matter in areas of the brain that dealt with memory, self-image, regulation of emotion and sense of perspective.

Other studies have shown increases in the hippocampus and frontal lobes.

Meditation may Decrease Sleep Requirements

Research conducted by the University of Kentucky showed that even novice meditators required fewer hours of sleep per night after meditating. The difference was more striking with experienced meditators. Meditation cannot replace all your sleep needs, but it can give you a boost if you need it

Simply put, meditation helps your brain work better. People who meditate on a regular basis report that they can concentrate more effectively and are able to work efficiently under stress.

Meditation Improves Focus and Attention

A University of California study shows that after meditation, participants were able to focus on dull and repetitive tasks more effectively.

With 20 minutes of meditation per day, students increased their cognitive skills by up to ten times. They were also able to perform better on stress-inducing timed tests.

Meditation helps to thicken the prefrontal cortex and can help stave off the loss of cognitive ability associated with old age.

Meditation Improves Information Processing

Long-term meditation practitioners show increased folding, or gyrification, of the cortex which indicates the brain has an increased ability to process information, and to process it faster. This allows people to make good decisions faster, form stronger memories and benefit from an increased attention span.

Meditation Decreases the Sensation of Pain

Researchers at the University of Montreal studied 26 participants, 13 Zen masters and 13 non-meditators. They exposed the participants to the same amount of pain-inducing heat and measured brain activity with an fMRI scanner. The Zen masters reported less pain, and their fMRI scans confirmed that they actually felt less pain.

In fact, in another study at the Wake Forest Baptist Medical Center meditation was shown to be more effective than morphine for pain control. After an hour of meditation training, participants reported a 40 percent reduction in pain intensity and a 57 percent reduction in the unpleasantness of pain. Morphine or other pain-relieving drugs typically reduce pain ratings by 25 percent.

Meditation Helps Manage ADHD

A study of 50 adult ADHD patients who had undergone mindfulness meditation training showed reduced hyperactivity, reduced impulsivity and an increased ability to act with awareness. This combination led to an overall improvement in ADHD symptoms.

Meditation Increases Focus, Even in Distracting Environments

Emory University researchers showed that participants in a study who had previously been trained in meditation showed increased connectivity in the attention-controlling areas of the brain. This helped the participants keep their focus and ignore distractions, even at times when they were not meditating.

Meditation Keeps You From Multitasking

Multitasking is a productivity myth. You may feel as though you are getting more work done but you aren't. Multitasking splits your attention and causes stress.

When a person attempts to multitask, they wind up feeling distracted and stressed.

Research conducted at the University of Washington and the University of Arizona with human resources personnel showed that those who practiced meditation reported lower levels of stress and had better memory when tested. They were able to focus on tasks for longer periods of time, decreasing the overall amount of time necessary for task completion.

Meditation Helps Allocate Brain Resources

When the brain is given two almost simultaneous tasks to concentrate on, the second is often unintentionally ignored. This effect is called attention blink. Research participants who spent three months of mindfulness meditation were able to decrease or eliminate their 'attention blink', allowing them to recognize both tasks. This shows less allocation of brain resources for each task, meaning they required less attention to focus and remember each task, not that they used less brain power to work on each task.

Meditation Improves Visual and Spatial Processing

With one to four sessions of mindfulness meditation training, working memory, executive function and visuospatial processing increased

Mindfulness Meditation Enhances Creativity

Research from Leiden University in The Netherlands showed that open monitoring meditation enhances creativity and the ability to think along new paths. Participants who participated in open monitoring meditation performed better than those who did not meditate when asked to develop new ideas.

Meditation and the Body

With all the benefits meditation provides for the brain and emotions, it is no surprise that meditation also benefits the physical body.

Meditation reduces the risk of heart disease and stroke

Heart disease is the largest killer in the world. In a 2012 study, 200 igh-risk participants were asked to take either a transcendental meditation class or a health education class geared toward a healthy diet and exercise routine. Over the next five years, researchers found that the participants who chose the transcendental meditation course had a 48 percent decrease in their risk of heart attack, stroke or death.

they noted that meditation "significantly reduced risk for mortality, myocardial infarction, and stroke in coronary heart disease patients. These changes were associated with lower blood pressure and psychosocial stress factors."

Meditation affects the expression of Stress and Immunity Genes

Harvard Medical School studies show that after practicing meditation and yoga, participants showed increased mitochondrial energy production, consumption and resiliency. This in turn provided the participants with higher immunity and resilience to stress.

Meditation Reduces Blood Pressure

Relaxation allows for the formation of nitric oxide, which opens the blood vessels. Research has shown that Zen meditation reduces blood pressure. Relaxation response meditation has shown 2/3 of participants with lowered blood pressure after three months. This resulted them requiring less medication.

Mindfulness and Inflammatory Disorders

Mindfulness meditation produces a wide variety of effects of patients, including reduced levels of pro-inflammatory genes, allowing participants to physically recover from a stress-inducing situation more quickly.

Meditation Helps You Live Longer

Data suggest that some forms of meditation helps stave off the shortening of telomeres (this is the basis of the aging process) by reducing stress arousal, cognitive stress and increasing positive states of mind and hormonal production.

Meditation and Personal Relationships

Now that meditation has helped our minds, emotions and bodies we are feeling quite good. It's no wonder that our interpersonal relationships will also improve.

Meditation Improves Empathy

The Buddhist practice of metta, or loving-kindness meditation, boosts people's ability to read facial expressions and empathize with others. Developing compassion increases the loving attitude one has for others, self-acceptance, social support and a general feeling of competence.

Metta Reduces Feelings of Social Isolation

A study published by the American Psychological Association reports that when participants spent just a few minutes in Metta meditation, they had increased feelings of positivity toward strangers, more feelings of social connection. This easily implemented technique increases positive social emotions and decreases feelings of isolation, even when people are still actually alone.

Science confirms the benefits practitioners of meditation have been espousing for centuries: Meditation promotes good health, prevents diseases, increases happiness, focuses concentration and allows you to feel more harmony throughout the world.

Misty Jordyn

CHAPTER FOURTEEN

THE CHAKRAS

Physics now tells us that matter is another form of energy. Our bodies are bundles of vibrating energies that make up patterns around our physical bodies.

One theory states that disease starts with disharmonious thoughts and emotional patterns. If these patterns persist, they block the natural flow of energy and begin to affect our physical bodies.

The chakra system is a system of nodes of energy that span the layers of energy bodies that connect with the physical body. The translation of energy between these layers is faster. There are seven major chakras, which correspond to the location of the major hormonal glands.

The first chakra, Muladhara, is located at the base of the spine, represents the physical identity and is associated with self-preservation. It represents the element earth and is related to our survival, our sense of grounding and the connection of our bodies to the physical plane. This chakra will bring us health, prosperity, security and a dynamic presence.

A simple exercise for the first chakra is: Stand with your feet about hip width apart, with your toes pointed toward each other just a bit. Press through your feet as though you were trying to push the floor apart. Inhale, bend your knees and exhale as you push down through your feet. Repeat this until your legs vibrate. This is a great exercise to do any time you find yourself standing in line, or even while talking on the phone.

The second chakra, Svadhisthana, is located in the abdomen, lower back and sexual organs, is associated with self-gratification and connects us to others through feeling, desire, sensation and movement. This chakra will bring grace, depth of feeling, sexual fulfillment and the ability to accept change.

A simple exercise for the second chakra is: Sit comfortably, legs crossed Indian style. Inhale, pushing the tip of your spine backward, opening the front of your sacrum, expanding and filling your lower belly. Imagine you are stretching your hips wide. Exhale, moving your sacrum in the opposite direction, pressing the navel back toward the spine. Repeat, building up speed as you go. Allow the fluidity of this pelvic movement to flow all the way up the spine.

The third chakra, Manipura, is located in the solar plexus, is associated with self-definition and rules our personal power and metabolism. When this chakra is healthy it brings energy, effectiveness, spontaneity and power.

A simple exercise for the third chakra is working in plank pose. Start by lying on the floor, face down. Place your hands below your shoulders, arms straight. Lift the entire body off the ground, toes curled under, body and legs one straight line, parallel to the floor. Hold for at least one minute. For added challenge balance on your forearms, elbows directly underneath the shoulders. For even more challenge, alternately lift each leg of the floor and hold.

The fourth chakra, Anahata, is the heart chakra and is in the middle of the seven. It is related to love and is the integrator of opposites in the psyche: mind and body, male and female, persona and shadow, ego and unity. A healthy fourth chakra allows us to love deeply, feel compassion, and have a deep sense of peace and centeredness.

A simple exercise for the fourth chakra is: Sit comfortably in a meditation posture. Straighten your spine, close your eyes and focus on your heart. Feel your heartbeat. Gently breathe in and out in a slow, steady rhythm. Imagine you are breathing in on the left side and expanding your heart out to the left. After a few breaths, imagine you are breathing from your right side and feel the right side of your heart expand. Now breathe into the bottom of your heart as you deepen your compassion for yourself and others. Finally, breathe into the top of your heart, lifting the heart to your shoulders pushing your energy out to the world.

The fifth chakra, Vishuddha, This is the chakra located in the throat and is thus related to communication and creativity. Here we experience the world symbolically through vibration, such as the vibration of sound representing language.

A simple exercise for the fifth chakra is: using the seed sounds of the chakras given in the ancient texts, called bija mantras. Repeat the sounds over and over at a rhythm that feels pleasant to you, going slow if you want to calm your chakras and faster if you want to stimulate them. You can sing them all in one tone, or you can go up in pitch with each chakra. Experiment to see what is most effective for you. The sounds are as follows: Chakra Sound 1 Lam 2 Vam 3 Ram 4 Yam 5 Ham 6 Ksham 7 Silence.

The sixth chakra, Ajna, is known as the brow chakra or third eye center. It is related to the act of seeing, both physically and intuitively. As such it opens our psychic faculties and our understanding of archetypal levels. When healthy it allows us to see clearly, in effect, letting us "see the big picture."

A simple exercise for the sixth chakra is: to "capture" light wherever you see it and bring it inside. Here's how you do it: Next time you are watching a beautiful sunset, open your entire awareness to the experience of drinking in the light. Then close your eyes and visualize what you just saw in your inner third eye. Keep doing it until you can call up the image at will. You can do this any time you see a particularly beautiful color, the glare of light coming off a car windshield, the way light plays on the trees as the breeze blows, the light of a candle during your meditation. See if you can retain these images that you bring inside, calling them up at will days later. This will help develop your third eye capacity.

The final chakra, Sahasrara, is the crown chakra that relates to consciousness as pure awareness. It is our connection to the greater world beyond, to a timeless, spaceless place of all-knowing. When developed, this chakra brings us knowledge, wisdom, understanding, spiritual connection, and bliss.

A simple exercise for the seventh chakra is: meditation. You can meditate while walking, focus on the breath, utter a mantra, imagine an image, or simply empty your mind completely and sit in emptiness. (That takes PRACTICE!). What is most important is to connect through the crown chakra to the limitless source, so that you are an open system, pulling that source into your crown and down through all your chakras. Opening the crown chakra is not just a matter of lifting our energy UP, but of moving it DOWN to manifestation as well. In this way the chakras become condensers of the cosmic energy of universal consciousness, condensing it into the seven levels of manifestation: thought, light, sound, air, fire, water, and earth.

A study of the chakras is beyond the scope of this book, but we will discuss them a bit more in Chapter 7, Magnetism and Auras.

Exercise to Open the Third Eye

With your eyes closed, envision your third eye area which is your brow chakra, just above and between your two eyes. Feel how open this area is and try to assign it a percentage. If it's not very open, imagine it opening a bit more, perhaps 10 or 20 percent more. Open and close it gently and see what feels comfortable.

Exercise to Adjust your Chakras

Visualize your chakras, one at a time from the root chakra at the base of the spine all the way up to the crown chakra at the top of the head. Pause at each chakra, seeing the front and back of each one. Imagine each chakra opening and closing, similar to the previous exercise. Set each chakra where it is comfortable for you before moving on. When you finish with the crown chakra, feel your entire body centered and balanced, all the chakras working in perfect alignment to transmit energy freely throughout your body.

Misty Jordyn

CONCLUSION

Yoga is an underutilized asset in our modern, busy world. It's a shame because just a few minutes, or even half a lunch break can make such a difference in the productivity and lives of almost everyone we know.

Deep breathing can work as an instant energy booster.

Meditation relaxes the overworked mind and overstressed body.

Alternate nose breathing allows for creative problem solving and clear thinking.

Yoga strengthen the body and mind, allowing the mind to be alert but relaxed, able to utilize intuition (our unconscious knowledge) more fully.

You have everything you need to reach all the goals you set for yourself in life, no matter how large they are. Set large goals, focus your intention and go for it. The strong body and clear mind that comes from a consistent practice of yoga can take you anywhere.

Misty Jordyn

൦൦൦FREE BONUS൦൦൦

Receive a **FREE Bonus Guide** to Jump Start healthy habits and sustain a *happy and healthy* lifestyle!

visit: http://bit.ly/1PoSRtE